Cardiac Effects of Hypothyroidism and Hyperthyroidism

Heart Problems caused by Thyroid Disease

By: James M. Lowrance © 2012

TABLE OF CONTENTS:

INTRODUCTION:

Thyroid disease is a major contributor to heart conditions of various types and can manifest as either hypothyroid or hyperthyroid disorders. This is why it is very important for both men and women (especially women), to be checked for abnormal thyroid hormone levels, beginning at age 35. A check for developing hypothyroidism or hyperthyroidism should also be done, at any point in life regardless of age, when symptoms of either condition appear to be developing.

Catching and treating thyroid disorders at their earliest stages, can help to prevent associated heart conditions from also developing or from worsening if already present. When people become thyroid hormone imbalanced, this can also exacerbate an already existing cardiac condition, which also means that treatments determined to be needed, by a qualified medical doctor or doctors (plural in cases when both an endocrinologist and cardiologist are needed), require more diligence on the part of both patient and physician, in order to extend life-expectancy and to maintain a better quality of life.

Within the chapters that follow, I will be addressing the types of heart conditions or cardiac effects that thyroid diseases can have on those who experience them. I will also discuss the treatments in-general, that are administered to correct or to help control these potentially serious problems. It is my sincere hope that this resource helps to provide a worthy general educational resource for its readers.

-Jim Lowrance

CHAPTER ONE

Hypercholesterolemia from Underactive Thyroid Gland

Hypothyroidism is the second leading cause of high cholesterol (Hypercholesterolemia), second-only to bad diet practices. This fatty substance that is found in the body, is actually a necessary type of fat molecule, that keeps tissues healthy throughout the body, when present at the proper levels (i.e. not too high and not too low, depending on the type being referenced).

Cholesterol Aids in the Manufacture of Steroid Hormones

This essential fat molecule is also the substance that helps convert adrenal hormones into other needed steroid hormones (sterones), including those that moderate sexual identity and functions. Without the needed manufactured hormones that result from conversion of them, via cholesterol, there would also be a problem with sodium and water balance in the body, the immune system could not operate properly and inflammation could not be moderated in the body without the aid of this essential precursor element.

Without its help, stress hormones (the major one being "cortical") would also not be present to keep the body from succumbing to chronic or traumatic stressors and experiencing even mild stress would become intolerable both mentally and physically.

Conversion of Sunlight into Vitamin D

Another steroid hormone of great importance, that could not be manufactured for use in the body without cholesterol, is "vitamin D", which was only recently recognized for its steroid effect, in addition to its value as a vitamin. Cholesterol is the substance that converts sunlight into vitamin D in the body as well, to be used for keeping bones, muscles and nerves healthy. Of course we also receive the nutrient from foods we consume but medical research has recently found that both proper diet and ample sunlight may not even be enough to boost proper levels of the nutrient within the body and so supplementation with the vitamin may also be necessary for many individuals. Without the aid of cholesterol however, vitamin D would have to be mega-supplemented as a lifelong practice.

High Cholesterol and Atherosclerosis

While the previously described positive effects, result from proper good cholesterol levels in the body, when the bad type becomes abnormally elevated, it can begin to stick to the walls of the arteries, throughout the body, as a type of "plaque". This is a condition referred to as "atherosclerosis" and the resulting effect of this condition includes a narrowing of blood flow through affected arteries and a hardening of them. If arteries leading to the heart become severely narrowed or completely blocked, this can result in a heart attack or heart failure and most-often in hypertension (high blood pressure) in its early stages. If the arteries leading from the heart to other parts of the body become affected, this can cause tissues starved of proper blood-nourishment, to become inoperable (paralyzed), including the arms or legs, which can be the result of a condition referred to as "Peripheral Artery Disease" (PAD), often beginning as a painful malady, that can also result in dangerous blood-clotting. When atherosclerosis from hypercholesterolemia results in loss of blood supply to the brain.

This is due to major arteries supplying blood to the organ being blocked, a stroke can be the result. In worse case scenarios, heart attacks and strokes can be fatal or can leave the afflicted person in a brain-vegetated state. Even in milder cases, a person can be left with varied degrees of brain damage and/or heart damage/failure.

Lipid Screenings and Thyroid Panels

These facts demonstrate the importance in regular lipid screenings (blood tests), to check for imbalances of either too-high a level of the cholesterol that can become bad for the body ("LDL" - low density lipoproteins) and/or too-low a level of the type that is good for the body ("HDL" - high density lipoproteins). This becomes more important when men and women reach ages 35 and older. If hypercholesterolemia is diagnosed (high LDL), it also becomes important to find the cause of the condition, so that it can be corrected to the fullest-extent (i.e. determining if there are contributing disorders, such as thyroid disease needing treatment).

In many cases an underlying cause may seem obvious, such as apparent morbid obesity.

Weight gain however, can be the result of hypothyroidism, as well as the cause of high cholesterol. With this being the case, blood testing of thyroid hormone levels should also be ordered, rather than taking-for-granted that the cause of imbalanced lipid levels is already apparent. A grouping of blood tests called a"thyroid panel" can be ordered with the simple stroke-of-a-pen by a doctor, to rule-out or to confirm thyroid involvement. While some patients in-whom a thyroid disease is missed due to a lack of testing, can actually see improvement in their hypercholesterolemia by being prescribed a medication for the condition called a "statin drug" (HMG-CoA reductase inhibitor), this would not correct the underlying hypothyroidism or the other harmful effects that can result from it over time. Treatment specifically for the underactive thyroid would also be necessary, to prevent further serious health consequences.

Hypothyroidism an Elusive cause of Hypercholesterolemia (Medical Research)

Following is a quote from medical research published on the PubMed website (U.S. National Institutes of Health).

Cardiac Effects of Hypothyroidism and Hyperthyroidism

He study is in regard to hypothyroidism not always being an apparent/obvious cause of hyperchortisolemia:

"Hypothyroidism is a cause of secondary hyperlipidaemia. This study investigates the frequency of biochemically diagnosed hypothyroidism and its relationship with plasma cholesterol concentration in apparently healthy people.

Thyroid function tests (total T4, TSH, and free T4) were performed on 272 apparently healthy men and women (179 vegetarians, 93 meat eaters) with a plasma cholesterol concentration above 7 mmol/l and on 90 individuals with a plasma cholesterol below 4.1 mmol/l who were matched for age, sex and dietary habits.

Six per cent of those with a plasma cholesterol above 7 mmol/l had biochemical evidence of hypothyroidism as defined by a TSH greater than 10 mIU/l (reference range 1-6) and a low free T4 below 10pmol/l (reference range 10.1-25).

Eighty per cent of these people had a high titre of thyroid anti-microsomal antibodies. Of the 90 individuals with a plasma cholesterol level below 4.1 and the 25 randomly selected participants none had biochemical evidence of hypothyroidism.

Hypothyroidism is relatively common in apparently healthy people with a raised plasma cholesterol. It appears no commoner in vegetarians than in meat eaters."

(From the Article Titled: "**Asymptomatic hypothyroidism and hypercholesterolaemia.**" - Online Link Location: http://www.ncbi.nlm.nih.gov/pmc/articles/PMC1293411/

Treating High Cholesterol in Hypothyroid Patients

In many cases of only mild to moderately elevated cholesterol in a newly diagnosed hypothyroid patient, treatment by their doctor, with thyroid hormone replacement therapy will resolve the issue once the hormones reach adequate and preferably "optimal levels" (suppressing TSH and raising T4 and T3 levels into the higher range of normal).

NOTE: "TSH" is a pituitary hormone that elevates with hypothyroidism, while the "T4 and T3" levels are the actual thyroid hormones that do the opposite of TSH and drop below normal with an underactive thyroid. The goal of hypothyroid treatment is to return each of these back to best-possible normal ranges.

If however, the cholesterol elevation is severe and/or a patient is also significantly obese or suffers from another endocrine disorder such as diabetes, other treatments may also be required, such as a prescribed statin drug as mentioned previously. Lifestyle changes would also likely be recommended by a treating doctor as well, even with normalized cholesterol levels, such as avoidance of a high-fat diet or one that indulges in the consumption of too much refined sugar (the manufactured types, that can highly increase triglycerides) and an increase in healthy foods that contain high-fiber content (i.e. fruits, vegetables, nuts and grains).

An increase in physical activity, such as a well-tolerated aerobic exercises would likely also be recommended (i.e. walking, jogging or bicycling).

Encouraging patients to practice stress-reduction methods might also be an added feature of treatment, due to the opinion by some medical experts, that high stress levels can actually contribute to increased bad cholesterol in the body. Highly activated stress hormones, can cause low reserves of them over time, leaving the body vulnerable to inflammation and an increase in fat storage by the body as it senses a chronic stress emergency (some sources refer to this as "adrenal fatigue"). Patients who smoke might be referred to programs to help them quit, since smoking can directly, negatively affect cholesterol metabolism in the body.

If the good "HDL" cholesterol level in a patient has dropped below normal, a doctor might also recommend that they take a daily fish oil supplement (a source of omega-3 fatty acids), which acts like the mechanism of good cholesterol, by helping to clear any excess LDL level from the arteries, thereby returning it to the liver, to be flushed as waste from the body. While cholesterol is essential to the body, it is important to keep both the good and bad levels of it, as well-balanced as possible for a healthier life.

Cardiac Effects of Hypothyroidism and Hyperthyroidism

CHAPTER TWO

Thyrotoxicity and Heart Arrhythmias

To become "thyrotoxic", can mean a number of things but a general understanding of the term would be "hyperthyroidism" (excessive thyroid hormone).

Causes of Thyrotoxicity

In most cases of thyrotoxicity, the cause is a disease process within the thyroid gland, such as the autoimmune condition called "Graves' disease" (over 90% of cases) or the development of tumors within the gland called "thyroid nodules" and more specifically those referred to as "hot nodules", which manufacture thyroid hormone just as natural thyroid tissue does but at abnormally high amounts. People can become overcharged with thyroid hormones for other reasons as well, including that which results from taking doses of thyroid hormone replacement (therapy for hypothyroidism), at excessively high amounts or due to over-supplementing with iodine that is an ingredient in a medication or in a natural supplement.

This can also include the consumption of large amounts of high-iodine content foods such as kelp (a type of seaweed - 1 tablespoon contains about 2000/mcg of iodine).

Manifestations of Being Thyrotoxic

The resulting effect of hyperthyroidism, is a bodily metabolism that is sped up to an abnormally high level. This will cause the person experiencing it, to feel high energy levels because the body will burn fuel coming into it (foods consumed), at an excessive rate. When this occurs, the following symptoms may result as shown below (some people will experience only some of these, depending on how severe the hyperthyroidism/thyrotoxicity is).

- Very high energy levels
- Diarrhea
- Anxiety and nervousness
- Increased Sweating
- Insomnia
- Hyperventilation (over-breathing) ...

- Hypertension (high blood pressure)
- Tachycardia episodes (spells of rapid heart rate)
- Muscle wasting
- Lack of nutrient retention (from chronic diarrhea)
- Bone loss (osteoporosis)

Two of the symptoms listed above (hypertension and tachycardia episodes), are the ones that have an effect on heart rhythm. Hypertension is a known cause for triggering abnormal heart beats over time but even apart from the high blood pressure, the person experiencing a hyperthyroid condition will experience episodes of tachycardia. When these two symptoms are combined, this increases the chances for the tachycardia to evolve into more serious types of chronic (sustained) heart arrhythmias, such as "Super Ventricular Tachycardia" (SVT), which originates from the lower chambers of the heart and "Paroxysmal Atrial Tachycardia" (PAT), which originates from the upper chambers of the heart.

If treatment to control or to resolve the thyrotoxicity is not administered and is allowed to continue, potentially fatal heart arrhythmias can eventually occur (rare), such as "Atrial Fibrillation" (more common and not usually life threatening) or "Ventricular Fibrillation" (episodes can cause fainting or sudden, fatal cardiac arrest). As SVT and/or PAT occur, a person may experience the symptoms listed, following.

- Angina (chest pain)
- Palpitations (strong sensations of heart beat)
- Dizziness
- Shortness of breath
- Sweating
- Syncope (fainting or near fainting)

Treatments for Thyrotoxicity

In order to control or to resolve heart arrhythmias caused by thyrotoxic conditions, the excessive levels of thyroid hormone in the body will need to be lowered back down into the normal range to restore a proper level of bodily metabolism.

If excessive iodine or oral thyroid hormone is the culprit, simply reducing or eliminating these, can resolve the heart palpitations and arrhythmias that are occurring. If a prescribed medication is involved, this will require the supervision of a medical doctor who can adjust a patient's dose, prescribe an alternative drug or add a new prescription to control this side effect, when a prescribed medication is mandatory and not able to be changed or stopped.

When hyperthyroidism caused by a condition such as Graves' disease is present, a doctor may prescribe one of a number of different anti-thyroid drugs ("thionamides" - those that lower thyroid hormone production). This would include drugs such as Methimazole (MMI) and Propylthiouracil (PTU). Another drug that may be prescribed, to control hypertension and tachycardia is a "beta-blocker", which reduces the effects of adrenaline on the cardiovascular system and may include brands such as Atenolol or Metoprolol.

Some hyperthyroid patients require a combination of both a beta-blocker and an anti-thyroid drug.

When a doctor determines that a diseased thyroid gland will not be controlled well-enough through medication treatment alone, he may refer a patient to a thyroid surgeon for removal of their gland (total thyroidectomy) or partial removal of their gland (sub-total thyroidectomy). A partial removal is usually the case when only one lobe of the gland is affected by a hot nodule, while total removal is often the case with Graves' disease patients (another term for the disease is "toxic diffuse goiter" - meaning the entire gland is affected). Another option however, is for the patient's gland to be "ablated", meaning it is destroyed via radioactive iodine, that is administered to the patient at a high-enough dose to fully eradicate all thyroid tissue from the body ("RAI" - Radioactive Iodine Ablation).

Treatment also becomes a priority due to tachycardia and other heart arrhythmias posing a risk for the development of an enlarged heart (Chronic Heart Failure) and/or a heart attack. In many cases, resolving the thyrotoxicity gives the heart opportunity to partially or fully recover from any enlargement or damage it has experienced.

Following is a PubMed medical research article quote, stating that atrial fibrillation is the most common type of heart arrhythmia associated with throtoxicity:

BACKGROUND:

Cardiac arrhythmias associated with thyrotoxicosis tend to be supraventricular in nature with atrial fibrillation being the most common. Ventricular arrhythmias are rarely associated with thyrotoxicosis and are considered to be secondary to intrinsic cardiac disease.

SUMMARY:

We present three patients with thyrotoxicosis and stable coronary disease in whom the primary cardiac rhythm disturbance was ventricular tachycardia. In all of these patients, the ventricular arrhythmias terminated with achievement of a euthyroid state. We hypothesize that the thyrotoxic state contributed to the etiology of, or lowered the threshold for the ventricular arrhythmias.

CONCLUSION:

Prompt attention to the management of thyrotoxicosis in patients with a history of significant heart disease is warranted in order to avoid potentially fatal arrhythmias.

(From the Article Titled: "**Thyrotoxicosis-induced ventricular arrhythmias.**" - Online Link Location: http://www.ncbi.nlm.nih.gov/pubmed/18816176)

Keep in mind when considering the facts stated in the above-quoted medical research, that tachycardia (rapid heartbeat) is very common with hyperthyroid conditions but it is not always considered an arrhythmia in the same sense as those described within the article. Tachycardia is also very common in other conditions such as anxiety disorders however, chronic anxiety or panic attacks do not cause a sustained type of severe tachycardia and seldom lead to actual heart conditions.

A resting heart rate above 100 beats per minute is determined to be higher-than-normal, whether sustained or intermittent.

This type of problem is often called a "palpitation" however, severe tachycardia that is prolonged (chronic), such as that occurring with untreated thyrotoxic states, can eventually lead to cardiomyopathy (heart failure) and enlargement of the heart as the valves within it, begin to stretch excessively due to the added strain placed upon them (valvular heart disease).This is why treating hyperthyroidism as early as possible, becomes important.

CHAPTER THREE

Hyperthyroid and Hypothyroid Cardiomyopathy

Within the previous chapters, reference was made to "cardiomyopathy" and "heart enlargement" however, while these conditions are often directly associated with each other, they are actually two different things.

What is Cardiomyopathy?

Cardiomyopathy actually is a term simply meaning that the heart muscle has become weakened for whatever reason, whether it be due to a disease process, chronic lack of oxygen or extremely strenuous activity placed upon the heart muscle. If for example, in a disease process, there is a connective-tissue disorder occurring within the body, such as Systemic Lupus Erythematosus ("SLE"- a body wide autoimmune condition), the heart can eventually become affected, leading to a weakening of the organ (this can also be true in some cases of Rheumatoid Arthritis and Sjögren's Syndrome).

If the scenario of prolonged hypoxia has occurred, meaning lack of oxygen in the body, such as that which occurs in people suffering from pulmonary (lung) disorders, this can eventually lead to cardiomyopathy as well (i.e. types of COPD, Lung Fibrosis and Lung Cancer).

If yet another scenario occurs, such as athletes who extend, excessively-added strain on the heart (beyond healthy levels) their hearts can eventually become weakened, rather than strengthened because they have gone beyond the muscle's tolerance level for extended periods of time. This has been reported to happen to pro football and basketball players, and to pro wrestlers, who have over-trained their bodies for many years, to reach peak performance and appearance levels however, their hearts were not given time to rest and repair and so they eventually became weakened as a result. This has also been found to be the case in athletes who have taken anabolic steroids to increase muscle size and strength, which placed undue strain on the heart muscle, leading to eventual cardiomyopathy.

The symptoms of cardiomyopathy may include the following:

- Fatigue and easy fatigability
- Shortness of breath
- Chest pain or discomfort
- Cardiac arrhythmias and/or palpitations

What is Heart Enlargement?

In the case of heart enlargement, the muscle expands to sizes that are outside of normal values, which can be due to a number of reasons as well. A major cause of heart enlargement however, is cardiomyopathy because when the heart weakens, it has to work harder to perform the same task of supplying blood-flow to every part of the body. Other causes or contributing-factors for heart enlargement, also referred to as "Chronic Heart Failure" (CHF), can include the following, as listed below.

- Diseases affecting heart valves (including severe Mitral Valve Prolapse)
- Severe untreated hypertension ...

- Heart damage (i.e. heart attack)
- Chronic Anemia
- Iron excess (hemochromatosis)
- Congenital heart defects (problems at birth)
- Morbid obesity
- Cigarette smoking
- Metabolic diseases (i.e. thyroid and diabetic disorders)

As this struggle with the heart continues, the heart attempts to compensate by widening its valves, which causes them to stretch. If this stretching of the heart is caught early enough, it can actually be reversed in some cases however, like a rubber band that only has so much elasticity, the valves and muscle can become stretched to the point that the enlargement cannot be reversed or can only be partially reversed. At this point, a treating doctor will attempt to halt further enlargement from occurring or to at least slow it down as much as possible.

When the heart enlarges, the same symptoms can occur that were listed previously for cardiomyopathy however, as the enlargement progresses, other symptoms, such as fluid retention in parts of the body ("edema" - swelling) will occur, most-often beginning in the feet and lower-legs but that can also manifest in the mid-section of the body and in the hands.

Patients with CHF may also develop breathing difficulties, such as asthmatic symptoms (cardiac asthma) and difficulty breathing after becoming supine for several minutes or hours ("orthopnea" - shortness of breath when laying flat). They may also hear noticeable wheezing or bubbling sounds coming from their lungs at times, which is caused by pulmonary edema (lung fluid) that builds within breathing passages.

Diagnosis and Treatments for Cadiomyopathy and Heart Enlargement

A doctor may suspect that his patient has myopathy or enlargement of their heart, if any of the symptoms listed previously are occurring. The patient would then be referred for cardiac testing, such as an"electrocardiogram".

This is also known as "EKG" and possibly the "stress test" version would be conducted, with observation during exertion and an "echocardiogram" (cardiac sonogram), which is a detailed sound-wave imaging of the heart, observed on a screen to monitor its functioning. In many cases, a typical chest x-ray (radiograph still image), will show any enlargement affecting certain valve-areas or of the heart in general.

A particular blood test that has been recently recognized as being <u>very accurate</u> for detecting even mild heart enlargement, is one called the "B-type Natriuretic Peptide" ("BNP" - a hormone released fromlower chambers of the heart if it experiences abnormal pressures). The test, according to some medical sources, is up to 98% accurate in detecting CHF and the upper-normal, cut-off value is "**<100 pg/ml**", meaning any results of the blood test that yield a result at 100 and above, are strongly indicative of heart failure/enlargement. Some abnormal values charts published by medical sources, state that readings between 100 and 300 indicate mild CHF, readings between 300 and 600 indicate moderate cases.

Those that are above 600, indicate severe heart failure (some patients see readings in the 1,000s).

The main focus when cardiomyopathy and/or heart enlargement is found, is to determine any underlying causes in order to treat them for control or elimination of them. This of course would include correcting thyrotoxic/hyperthyroid states, which will lift the excessive pressure from the heart, allowing it a degree of rest and repair (possible complete reversal). In addition to eliminating contributing factors to also include cessation of smoking and weight loss for obese patients, other things added to a treatment regimen by a patient's doctor, may include the following.

- Regular exercise at proper tolerance level
- A healthy diet
- Reduced fluid intake
- Removing sodium from the diet (salt – which results in fluid retention)
- Hypertensive medications

Following is a PubMed medical research article, that refers to "idiopathic dilated cardiomyopathy", as related to thyroid disorders.

"Severe thyrotoxicosis can cause irreversible congestive heart failure. To investigate the coincidence of subclinical thyroid disorders and idiopathic dilated cardiomyopathy (IDC) we investigated these patients with respect to their morphological and functional thyroid status. Thyroid sonography as well as thyroid hormone levels were measured in all patients.

RESULTS: Sixty-one patients (50 male, 11 female) with chronic stable IDC were included. Two out of 61 patients showed completely normal thyroid morphology and function. The other 59 patients showed either morphological or functional abnormalities or both. Of the 53 patients with morphological abnormalities 23 patients (all male) showed diffuse goiter as opposed to 29 nodular enlarged organs (24 male, 5 female). No clinically significant hypothyroidism or thyrotoxicosis was seen. A good correlation was found between the duration of IDC and thyroid volume ($r = 0.44$; $p < 0.001$).

Two patients died during the study period, 1 from sudden death and 1 from progressive heart failure.

CONCLUSION: Subclinical thyroid disorders are frequently seen in patients with long-standing IDC when they live in an area of chronic iodine deficiency. This can be explained by chronic salt restriction as basic treatment for congestive heart failure. Therefore we conclude that examination of the thyroid gland should be done routinely in patients with IDC, especially when restriction of salt intake is recommended by the treating physician."

(From the Article Titled: **"Subclinical thyroid disorders in patients with dilated cardiomyopathy."** - Online Link Location: http://www.ncbi.nlm.nih.gov/pubmed/9096916)

The preceding information clearly conveys the importance in getting thyrotoxic states normalized to prevent these types of cardiac issues from occurring or worsening.

CHAPTER FOUR

PVCs and PACs from Thyroid Hormone Imbalance

Premature Ventricular Contractions (PVCs) and Premature Atrial Contractions (PACs) are also referred to as "ectopic heartbeats".

What are PVCs and PACs and Why do They Occur?

These common and usually benign heart arrhythmias (also referred to as "dysrhythmias") are extra beats that are triggered by cells within the heart-muscle, located close to the lower chambers of the heart (the ventricles) or close to the upper chambers (the atria), that become excitable/charged with the ability to emit mild electrical impulses.

The heart normally beats as a result of its own electrical pacemaker system but the extra electrical impulses that occur with PVCs and PACs, actually add extra beats in-between those the natural pacemaker is already triggering.

Symptoms of Ectopic Heartbeats

In spite of these being extra beats, they will feel more like pauses in the heartbeat to the person who experiences them. After the pause-sensation, some people who experience ectopic heartbeats, also describe the feeling of an extra-hard beat following it, or what they might call a strong thump inside their chest. This is due to the very slightly added extra-time of only a second or two for the heart to fill-up with blood, so that when it fully contracts, there is slightly more blood being pushed-out. These sensations, that can also include feelings such as the heart fluttering, flip-flopping, pounding or slightly changing speeds, also places them in the "palpitations" category.

Some people with ectopic beats may report these other symptoms occurring with them as well:

- Anxiety or panic feelings
- Mild adrenaline surges
- Slight dizziness
- Minor chest pain or discomfort
- Head rush (sudden blush) ...

- Urge to cough
- Shortness of breath
- Mild headaches
- Insomnia

While PVCs and PACs are harmless in the vast majority of cases, some can be associated with serious heart conditions and should be evaluated by a medical doctor, as a precaution. This is especially true, if any of the symptoms listed-above become significant or if a patient has a past history of significant heart problems. Most patients can be given the clear by their doctor, with a simple physical evaluation but if there is any suspicion for structural heart damage or abnormalities, a patient might be referred to a cardiologist or for diagnostic testing such as an EKG or echocardiogram.

Some patients presenting with a variety of different palpitations, are discovered to have a common "click heart murmur" called "Mitral Valve Prolapse" ("MVP" - briefly referenced earlier in a list of possible causes for heart enlargement).

The condition is common in the general population and slightly more common in thyroid patients but in the vast majority of cases it is benign and requires only lifestyle changes or a beta-blocker drug to help control any symptoms it is causing. In severe cases of MVP, in which significant "mitral regurgitation" is present, surgery may be required to repair the faulty heart valve (rare). Otherwise, MVP-Syndrome (the "syndrome" suffix added when symptoms are present), is simply a condition that can be an annoyance to some patients but is rarely ever life-threatening and very seldom requires surgical intervention. The condition can however, cause or contribute to the frequency of PVCs and/or PACs in people who experience it.

Ectopic Beats Caused by Thyroid Hormone Imbalance

Among the causes of PVCs and PACS, are included things such as stress and anxiety, lack of sleep, intake of stimulants (i.e. tobacco, alcohol, caffeine and refined-sugar excess), increased exercise (during or following) and hormonal imbalances.

Women report that ectopic beats can correlate with their menstrual cycles and pregnancies, and certainly with added stressors of any kind, the body can be flooded with more adrenal hormones (catecholamines). Another cause however, that has been reported by those who experience these palpitations that can be very annoying and sometimes very concerning to those who experience them, is "thyroid hormone imbalance".

While it is understandable that hyperthyroid patients would experience these, with the added adrenaline in their bodies resulting from thyrotoxicity, patients with hypothyroidism also report experiencing them.

It's very possible that either abnormally low or abnormally high levels of hormones that are of any endocrine type (i.e. thyroid, adrenal, glucose regulating and the sex types), can potentially cause episodes of these added heartbeats. This can be true of natural hormones within the body that fluctuate and true of supplemented hormones, coming into the body from an outside source, if fluctuations in them occur as well.

Avoiding the Added Heartbeats as a Thyroid Patient

With hormones apparently playing a factor in these sometimes scary palpitations, one should not only avoid the triggers listed previously, such as added stressors, sleep deprivation and consuming too many stimulants (i.e. caffeinated coffee/tea, alcoholic beverages and manufactured sugars), one should also attempt to keep their hormones properly balanced as best possible. This would include thyroid hormones that are being taken as replacement therapy for hypothyroidism. In order to accomplish this, hypothyroid patients should report any symptom-changes in their treated underactive thyroid conditions, to their doctors, in case a new blood test needs ordered sooner than scheduled to determine if a dose-change in the therapy is needed. The daily dose prescribed should be taken faithfully, usually first thing in the morning on an empty stomach (at least 30 minutes before eating), with plenty of water to help it absorb into the system. Any supplements or foods with high calcium or any iron in them, should not be consumed until 6 hours after a thyroid dose is ingested (these can hinder its absorption).

While some patients develop hypothyroidism as the direct result of a disease within their glands, others develop it as the expected after-effect of treatments for hyperthyroidism (i.e. following thyroidectomies or RAI ablations). Either way, thyroid hormone replacement therapy is the required life-long treatment, for which there is no alternative.

Patients whose hypothyroid therapies are well-regulated as reflected by optimal normal-values blood test results of their TSH, T3 and T4 levels, only need retested, every 4 to 6 months once a euthyroid state is achieved (normalized metabolism). Testing may need to be repeated sooner however, if symptoms manifest between blood retests that are scheduled this far ahead and this should include the onset of heart palpitations of any type. Not only can ectopic heartbeats signal an abnormal change in thyroid hormone levels but other types of palpitations can as well, including tachycardia (possibly indicating over-treatment with thyroid hormone) and "bradycardia" (a slowed heart rate, possibly indicating under-treatment). NOTE: Bradycardia is defined as a resting heart rate of below 60 beats per minute.

Cardiac Effects of Hypothyroidism and Hyperthyroidism

If additional medical treatment is needed for heart palpitations, this will usually be a beta-blocker medication and lifestyle changes, as discussed within the previous chapters. There are different classes of"anti-arrhythmic drugs" available however, doctors usually prescribe these for the more serious types of heart arrhythmias rather than for ectopic beats which are usually not considered a risk-factor for anything potentially serious in otherwise heart-healthy individuals.

Some patients with serious types of arrhythmias are also referred to an electrophysiologist, which is a cardiologist who specializes in the electrical system of the heart. The specialist might then opt to perform what is referred-to as a "Radio frequency ablation" (RFA). This is a procedure in which a catheter, is inserted into the area of the heart where an arrhythmia originates-from and an electrode contained inside the catheter, transmits radio waves that ablate (destroy) a small area of heart tissue. This can stop the abnormal impulses being transmitted by the heart's natural pacemaker however, the procedure carries some risks and is very rarely recommended for people with benign PVCs and/or PACs.

Cardiac Effects of Hypothyroidism and Hyperthyroidism

Following is an interesting medical research study in regard to ectopic heartbeats associated with thyroid hormone replacement therapy (the thyroid hormone dose did not increase PVCs but did slightly increase PACs in some of the participants studied):

"Whether thyroid replacement therapy can trigger cardiac arrhythmias in patients with hypothyroidism is not known. In this prospective study, 24 h ambulatory electrocardiographic (ECG) monitoring was used to assess the frequency of atrial and ventricular premature beats in 25 patients with hypothyroidism (5 men and 20 women, aged 56 +/- 3 years) before and 3.5 +/- 0.5 months (mean +/- SEM) after thyroid replacement therapy. Plasma thyroid-stimulating hormone was 73.6 +/- 12.3 and 3.1 +/- 0.6 microU/ml and free thyroxine index was 2.4 +/- 0.4 and 9.8 +/- 0.9 micrograms/100 ml at baseline and after thyroid replacement therapy, respectively.

...

The frequency of ventricular premature beats was not affected by thyroid replacement therapy (from 273 +/- 221 at baseline to 352 +/- 235 beats/24 h after therapy), even in patients with frequent baseline arrhythmias.

In contrast, the frequency of atrial premature beats was slightly increased after thyroid replacement therapy (from 47 +/- 17 to 279 +/- 197 beats/24 h), largely as a result of changes seen in three patients. No patient developed new onset of sustained ventricular or supraventricular arrhythmias.

Average, basal and maximal heart rates during ECG monitoring increased significantly after thyroid replacement therapy (average 72 +/- 2 to 80 +/- 2; basal 64 +/- 2 to 70 +/- 2; maximal 114 +/- 3 to 130 +/- 3 beats/min, respectively, p less than 0.001).

In conclusion, thyroid replacement therapy is safe in patients with common benign cardiac arrhythmias, and does not trigger an increase in arrhythmia frequency except in rare patients with baseline atrialpremature beats.

It is, however, associated with an increase in basal, average and maximal heart rates."

(From the Article Titled: **"Effect of thyroid replacement therapy on the frequency of benign atrial and ventricular arrhythmias"** - Online Link Location: http://www.ncbi.nlm.nih.gov/pubmed/2477427)

Conclusion:

It is my hope that the information contained within this chapter and those that preceded it, have provided helpful information to thyroid patients seeking a general education regarding the more common cardiac manifestations of thyroid disease. I offer "Best Wishes" to all of my fellow treated thyroid patients

(END)

About the Author:

I am a husband, father, grandfather and lifetime contract salesman, with experience in health writing that began in 2004. I completed theological studies with Liberty University in 1996. I formerly served as editor and forum moderator of Thyroid Health for a major multi-topic content site and as a general health writer for another, where I achieved Editor's Choice Awards for my articles on health subjects.

In 2003 I was diagnosed with hypothyroidism; "Hashimoto's thyroiditis" being the cause. This autoimmune form of thyroid disease that causes destruction of the thyroid gland resulted in my also developing "Chronic Fatigue Syndrome", due to a compromised immune system with severe co-morbid "Adrenal Fatigue". I also suffered severe anxiety symptoms, including panic attacks early into the onset of Hashimoto's thyroiditis (Hashitoxicosis) and clinical depression. I was also diagnosed with peripheral neuropathy and thyroid myopathy, with co-morbid nutritional deficiencies. I have also experienced episodic ectopic heartbeats, since my teen years, partially as a result of MVP-Syndrome.

My eventual receiving of diagnoses was a difficult process with proper diagnostic testing not being ordered by the first doctors I sought treatment from. These types of issues were inspiration for me to become proactive in my own health care and to self-educate myself on these health disorders, which I have done extensively since 2003. I now enjoy sharing this information with other patients experiencing my same health disorders.

www.ingramcontent.com/pod-product-compliance
Lightning Source LLC
Chambersburg PA
CBHW061229280526
45784CB00006B/2699

* 9 7 8 1 4 6 9 9 9 6 9 3 6 *